ASK WHY?

MEDICAL ETHICS 101

ASK WHY?

MEDICAL ETHICS 101

by

David A. Kent, M.D. Psychiatrist

Ask Why?: Medical Ethics 101
David A. Kent, M.D. Psychiatrist

Papereback Edition ISBN: 979-8-9937794-6-1
Ebook Edition ISBN: 979-8-9937794-7-8

www.davidkentauthor.com

Flames Creations | Design Services Provided by Flames Creations

CONTENTS

INTRODUCTION

Picture the phone ringing at 3 a.m.

You already know that isn't a good hour for a phone call. On the other end is a voice from a hospital, and in a single sentence your whole world tilts. Someone you love has been in an accident. Or a scan found something. Or a parent who was fine yesterday can no longer speak for themselves today.

Now the questions start coming at you, fast, from people in scrubs who are kind but in a hurry.

Do you want us to do everything we can?
What would she have wanted?
Who has the authority to decide?

And you realize, standing in that hallway, that you don't know. Not because you're careless, and not because you don't love the person in that bed. You don't know because no one ever taught you. No one sat you down and walked you through it.

Let me ask you a few of those questions now, while the room is quiet and no one is rushing you.

If you could not speak for yourself tomorrow, do you know who would speak for you? Would they actually know what you want — or would they be guessing, and quietly tearing themselves apart over the guess? If a doctor offered you a treatment, would you know how to ask whether it's truly worth it? If someone you love were seriously ill and refusing all help, do you know what you could actually do about it — or what the law would and would not allow? Would you know how to tell when more treatment has stopped helping and started hurting? Do you know the difference between a living will and a regular will? Between someone holding your power of attorney and a court appointing a guardian? Do you know where you'd even go to find honest medical information in a world that is drowning in bad advice?

If you don't have quick answers, you are not behind. You are simply human, and completely normal. We teach our kids how to drive a car and how to fill out a tax form. We almost never teach them how to make the hardest decisions of a human life — the ones about their own bodies, their own endings, and the people they'll leave to sort it all out.

That is the gap this book is here to close.

These pages are not written for doctors or lawyers. They're written for you — the daughter in the hallway, the husband holding the clipboard, the patient who nodded along in the appointment and didn't understand half of it, the parent trying to decide how much say a teenager should have. This is a plain-language guide to the moments when things go wrong, and to the choices those moments force on us.

You'll meet people in these pages. A woman who signs a form she doesn't understand. A mother who cannot get help for the grown son she is watching come apart. A daughter asked at midnight whether she wants the doctors to do everything. Their stories are composites — invented people, drawn from the kinds of situations that unfold in hospitals every single day. They are how this book explains itself: not with rules, but with people.

I believe a few things, and they run underneath every chapter.

I believe that good health, and a real say in your own care, is not a luxury for the well-informed. It is closer to a human right. I believe that when the hard moment comes, you deserve to have everything on the table — every option, every question, every consequence — spoken to you in words you can actually understand. And I believe there is no single "right" answer that fits everyone, because the right answer depends on who you are: what you believe, what you love, and what you can live with. The goal of this book is never to tell you what to choose. It's to make sure that when you choose, the choice is truly yours.

None of this is meant to frighten you. Fear is what happens when the hard questions arrive and we have no answers ready. The opposite of that fear is not pretending nothing bad will ever happen. The opposite is preparation. It's knowing the questions before they're asked of you. It's understanding your own wishes well enough to say them out loud, and to write them down, so that the people you love are never left guessing in a hallway at 3 a.m.

That is what knowledge gives you here: not certainty that nothing will go wrong, but control over how you meet it when it does. And there is something quietly powerful in that control. It's a gift you give yourself, and an even bigger gift you give the people who will one day have to speak for you.

So read this book slowly. Argue with it. Talk about it at the dinner table, uncomfortable as that sounds. Ask yourself the questions before life asks them for you.

Because the most important question in this entire book isn't a medical one. It's a human one.

And it begins with two words: *Ask why.*

Why do we choose what we choose? Why does it matter so much who decides? Why are we so rarely ready?

Let's find out together.

CHAPTER ONE

WHY DO TWO PEOPLE MAKE OPPOSITE CHOICES?

Ruth is sixty-two. She has raised four children, buried a husband, and taught third grade for thirty-one years. She sits in exam room 4 with her purse still in her lap, and when the doctor finishes explaining it all — the illness, the treatment, the odds, the months it will take — she doesn't hesitate for a second. "Yes," she says. "Let's get started."

James is also sixty-two. He spent his working life as a lineman for the power company, which means he spent it being careful for a living. He sits in exam room 7, thirty feet down the same hall, and hears the same doctor say very nearly the same words about the same illness. He listens all the way to the end. Then he says, "No. Thank you, but no." He picks up his jacket and drives home.

Same age. Same illness. Same treatment, offered by the same doctor, on the same Tuesday afternoon. Opposite answers.

Why?

That question is the heart of this whole book, and the answer is simpler than you'd think. Nobody walks into a doctor's office as a blank page.

We each bring a lifetime of invisible baggage with us. We can't see it, but it's in the room, and it shapes almost every choice we make about our health.

Three things fill that baggage more than anything else: what we believe, where we come from, and what happened to us when we were young. Our faith, our culture, and our childhood. Let's open each one up.

WHAT WE BELIEVE

For a lot of people, faith isn't a side topic. It's the lens they see everything through, including sickness and healing.

Some faiths teach that a person shouldn't accept blood from someone else, even to save their own life. Some have strong beliefs about the beginning of life, or birth control, or what should and shouldn't be done at the very end. Some see mental illness not as a medical problem at all, but as a spiritual struggle, something to pray through rather than treat with medicine.

Here's the important part, and it's easy to get wrong: this chapter is not about deciding whose beliefs are correct. It's about noticing that beliefs are *there*, sitting in the room, helping to steer the choice.

A good doctor learns to work *with* a patient's beliefs, not around them or against them. Pretending the beliefs don't exist doesn't make them go away. It just makes the patient feel unheard, and a patient who feels unheard often walks out the door.

Here's what working *with* a belief actually looks like.

A man — call him Daniel — needs an operation that would ordinarily involve a blood transfusion. His faith does not permit him to accept blood, and he says so at the first appointment, bracing for the argument he has had before.

It doesn't come. The surgeon asks questions instead. What exactly is and isn't permitted? Are there treatments in the gray area he'd want to think about? Who else does he want in the room when they talk it through?

Then the surgical team goes after the problem *as a problem.* They build a plan around it: medications for weeks beforehand to raise his own blood counts, surgical techniques that lose less blood, equipment that recycles and returns his own blood as they go. None of it crosses a line Daniel believes in. All of it is real medicine.

The surgery goes fine.

It doesn't always work out that neatly, and this book won't pretend otherwise — sometimes there's no workaround, and the conversation gets much harder. But notice what that surgeon did before any of the medicine started. He treated Daniel's belief as a *fact about the case* — a real constraint to plan around, like an allergy or a bad heart — rather than an obstacle to be talked out of.

The alternative would almost certainly have cost him his patient. Lectured, or quietly assumed to be someone who'd cave once he got scared enough, Daniel would have gone somewhere else. Or nowhere at all.

So when you see someone make a medical choice that surprises you, the first quiet question to ask is: what do they believe? The answer usually explains a lot.

WHERE WE COME FROM

Culture is the second piece of baggage, and it surprises people the most.

Imagine a family gets bad news about their grandmother. In much of the United States, the doctor tells the grandmother directly. We treat that as basic respect: it's her body, her life, her news to hear first.

Now picture a different family, raised somewhere with different customs. The doctor is expected to tell the *adult children* first. They decide together how much to tell grandmother, and sometimes they choose to protect her from the hardest details. To them, *that* is what love and respect look like. You don't lay a frightening burden on an elder. You carry it for her.

This isn't just an impression. Researchers have measured it. In one well-known study of older adults in Los Angeles, most European Americans and African Americans — around 87 to 88 percent — believed a patient should be told directly about a terminal diagnosis. But far fewer Korean Americans (47 percent) and Mexican Americans (65 percent) agreed. Many of them felt the family should receive the news and decide together how to handle it.[1] Neither group was confused about right and wrong. They simply started from different ideas about what caring for someone looks like.

So which family is right?

That's a trap question. Neither one is wrong. One puts the individual first. The other puts the family first. Both are trying to do right by the person they love.

Culture shapes more than just who hears the news. It shapes how people show pain, or hide it. Whether they want a room full of relatives or want to face things alone. How they think about death. Whether they'd feel comfortable with a doctor of a different gender examining them.

None of this shows up on a lab test. But it's in the room the whole time.

WHAT HAPPENED TO US YOUNG

The third piece of baggage is the quietest, and often the most powerful. It's childhood.

Think about your own first memories of doctors. Maybe you had a kind one, and the office felt safe. Or maybe you got a shot that hurt and nobody warned you, or you were sick and scared and felt like no one was listening. Maybe something painful happened that you've never really talked about.

Whatever it was, you didn't leave it behind in childhood. You carry it. We all do.

And this isn't just a feeling, either. In one of the largest studies of its kind, researchers at the Centers for Disease Control and Kaiser Permanente surveyed more than 17,000 adults about their childhoods. They found something striking: the more hard experiences a person had growing up — abuse, neglect, a home in chaos — the higher their risk of serious health problems decades later. The pattern was steady and clear. More hardship early meant more risk later.[2] And these experiences turned out to be far more common than anyone expected. About two out of three of those adults had lived through at least one of them.

So the grown-up who "hates doctors" and puts off every appointment often isn't being stubborn. Somewhere back there, a doctor's office taught them that it isn't a safe place. The person who won't take their medicine may have learned young not to trust anyone in charge. The patient who braces for the worst before the doctor even speaks may be reliving an old moment when the news really was that bad.

These early lessons run deep and quiet. Most people don't even know they're following them. They just feel a knot in the stomach in the waiting room and can't say why.

WHY THIS MATTERS TO YOU

So we come back to Ruth and James, thirty feet apart, saying yes and no to the same treatment. By now you can see that they were never really deciding with the same information at all. Ruth was hearing that doctor through a lifetime of faith that told her life is a gift worth fighting for. James was hearing him through the memory of his own father, who took a treatment much like this one and spent his last good months too sick to fish, too sick to talk, too sick to be himself. They brought different baggage, so they made different choices. And from the inside, both choices made perfect sense.

There are two takeaways here, and they're both useful the next time you or someone you love is sitting in that exam room.

First, for yourself: your reactions are not random, and they're not something to be ashamed of. They come from somewhere. If you can name your own baggage — *I don't trust hospitals because of what happened to my dad*, or *my faith shapes how I feel about this* — you can make a clearer choice, one that's actually yours instead of one your past is quietly making for you.

Second, for everyone else: when a person makes a health choice that looks strange or even foolish to you, hold off on the word "crazy." Nine times out of ten, there's a reason, and it's hiding in one of these three places — what they believe, where they come from, or what happened to them long ago.

The best doctors already work this way. They even have a name for it: *cultural humility*. It means treating each patient as the world's leading expert on their own life, and staying curious instead of assuming.[3] And here's the good news — you don't need a medical degree to do the same thing. Anyone can. A little curiosity, aimed at yourself and at the people you love, changes everything.

Because once you see the baggage, you can't unsee it. And you'll start asking a much better question than *"Why would anyone do that?"*

You'll start asking, *"What are they carrying?"*

That single shift — from judging to understanding — is where good medicine and good relationships both begin. It costs you nothing. It's available to you right now, in the very next hard conversation you have. And it turns a frightening, confusing moment into something gentler: two people, each carrying their own history, trying to find the right answer together.

That's not just better ethics. It's a kinder way to be human. And it's a very good place to begin.

NOTES

[1] Blackhall LJ, Murphy ST, Frank G, Michel V, Azen S. "Ethnicity and Attitudes Toward Patient Autonomy." *JAMA.* 1995;274(10):820–825.

[2] Felitti VJ, Anda RF, Nordenberg D, et al. "Relationship of Childhood Abuse and Household Dysfunction to Many of the Leading Causes of Death in Adults: The Adverse Childhood Experiences (ACE) Study." *American Journal of Preventive Medicine.* 1998;14(4):245–258.

[3] Tervalon M, Murray-García J. "Cultural Humility Versus Cultural Competence: A Critical Distinction in Defining Physician Training Outcomes in Multicultural Education." *Journal of Health Care for the Poor and Underserved.* 1998;9(2):117–125.

CHAPTER TWO
IT'S YOUR CHOICE — BUT DO YOU REALLY UNDERSTAND IT?

Maria is sitting on the edge of a hospital bed in a paper gown. Surgery is in an hour. A kind nurse hands her a clipboard with several pages on it and points to a line at the bottom. "Just your signature here, hon."

Maria signs. She always signs. The pages are full of long words — *anesthesia*, *complications*, *contraindications* — and she doesn't really understand them, but the doctor seems sure, everyone's busy, and she doesn't want to be difficult. So she writes her name, and a few minutes later someone wheels her away.

Did Maria just give informed consent?

Legally, maybe. Truly? No. And the gap between those two answers is one of the most important ideas in all of medicine.

A SIGNATURE IS NOT THE SAME AS UNDERSTANDING

We tend to think consent is a piece of paper. It isn't. The paper is just proof. The real thing — the thing that actually protects you — is *understanding*. Informed consent means you know what's about to happen to your body, you know what could go wrong, you know what else you could do instead, and *then* you agree.

Think of it like signing for a house. Nobody would sign a mortgage they hadn't read, on a house they'd never seen, just because the agent was in a hurry. Yet we do exactly that with our own bodies all the time — and the stakes are far higher than a house.

So what does real consent actually require? Doctors and ethicists usually break it into four plain pieces:

One: You're able to decide. You're awake, thinking clearly, and able to weigh a choice. (Later in the book we'll talk about what happens when someone can't — a child, or a person who's confused or unconscious.)

Two: You're told what you need to know. Not a medical lecture. Just the things that matter: what's wrong with you, what the treatment is, what good it's likely to do, what could go wrong, and — the part people forget — what your other options are, *including doing nothing at all.*

Three: You actually understand it. Not "the doctor said words." You could explain it back in your own kitchen to your sister.

Four: You're choosing freely. No one is rushing you, scaring you, or shaming you into it.

Notice that Maria only had one of the four. She could decide, sure. But she wasn't really told in plain words, she didn't understand, and she was gently pressured by the rush of the moment. One out of four is not consent. It's a signature.

IT WASN'T ALWAYS THIS WAY

Here's something that surprises most people: for most of human history, patients weren't asked at all.

For centuries, the doctor decided. The doctor often didn't even tell you what you had — especially if the news was bad. Keeping patients in the dark was considered *kind.* The idea that it was your body and therefore your call is, historically speaking, brand new.

The turning point in America came from the courts. In 1914, a judge named Benjamin Cardozo wrote a line that still echoes today: that every grown adult of sound mind has the right to decide what happens to his own body.[1] That was the seed. The actual phrase "informed consent" wasn't even born until a 1957 court case.[2] And the idea got its real teeth in 1972, in a case called *Canterbury v. Spence.* A young man had spinal surgery, was never warned it carried a risk of paralysis, and was left paralyzed. The court ruled that a doctor has a duty to tell you the risks a reasonable person would want to know — not just the ones the doctor feels like mentioning.[3]

In other words: the law now says the information belongs to *you.* It is not a gift the doctor chooses to give. It's yours by right.

WHY THIS IS HARDER THAN IT SOUNDS

If consent depends on understanding, we have a problem — because medicine is confusing on purpose. It has its own language, built over centuries, and it does not translate itself for you at the bedside.

How big is this problem? A major national survey found that only about 12 percent of American adults have what experts call "proficient" health literacy — the ability to comfortably read and use everyday health information. More than 77 million adults are at the "basic" or "below basic" level.[4] Read that again. It means that if you have ever felt lost, embarrassed, or overwhelmed in a doctor's office, *you are not the exception. You are the vast majority.*

This matters because it flips the blame. When a patient doesn't understand, that is not the patient's failure. It's a failure of explaining. And you are completely within your rights to say, "I need you to explain that again, in plain English."

THE MOST POWERFUL WORDS YOU OWN

So what do you actually do? You ask. Real consent is a conversation, and you're allowed to lead it. Here are the questions that unlock it — bring them written on a card if you need to:

What is actually wrong with me, in plain words?

What are my choices — *all* of them — including waiting or doing nothing?

What are the benefits and the risks of each choice?

How will this change my daily life?

What happens if I do nothing?

And then the single most useful trick of all, one that doctors themselves are taught to invite: **explain it back.** Say, "Let me make sure I've got this right," and repeat the plan in your own words. If you can't, you don't understand it yet — and that's exactly what you need to find out *before* you sign, not after.

One more thing, and it's important: saying yes is your right, but so is saying no. You are allowed to refuse. You are allowed to say "not yet." You are allowed to ask for a second opinion. A good doctor will not be offended by any of this. A good doctor will be relieved, because a patient who truly understands is a patient who heals better and trusts more.

WHAT HAPPENED TO MARIA

Maria's surgery went fine.

That's worth saying plainly, because the story people expect here is a disaster, and most of the time there isn't one. She healed. She went home. She was grateful.

What she learned six weeks later, at a follow-up, was that there had been another option — a smaller procedure with a longer recovery and less risk, which some patients in her situation choose instead. It might not have been right for her. She might well have picked the surgery anyway.

But she hadn't known it existed.

She wasn't angry about it. She said the thing so many patients say, in one form or another: *I didn't know I was allowed to ask.*

Fourteen months later, Maria is in a clinic again, this time about her knee, and someone hands her a clipboard. And this time she does something different. She holds onto it. She looks up and says, "Before I sign — can you walk me through this in plain words? What are all my choices, including doing nothing? And what happens if I wait six months?"

The physician assistant sits down.

That's the tell, by the way. When someone sits down, the conversation has changed. They talk for eleven minutes. Maria ends up choosing physical therapy first, with surgery held in reserve.

Maybe that turns out to be the right call, and maybe it doesn't — she'll find out. That isn't the point. The point is that this time, the decision was actually hers.

THE GOOD NEWS

Notice how small the change was.

Maria didn't get smarter between those two appointments. She didn't read a medical textbook or learn a word of Latin. She learned exactly one thing: that the clipboard was never a formality. It was an invitation.

That single realization turned her from a passenger into the driver. And here's the best part: it costs nothing, it requires no medical training, and it is available to every one of us, every single time.

That's the quiet power hiding inside informed consent. It isn't a form to sign. It's a right to understand — and a conversation you are always allowed to lead. You don't have to be the smartest person in the room. You just have to be willing to ask one more question.

And that, it turns out, is something anyone can do.

NOTES

[1] *Schloendorff v. Society of New York Hospital*, 211 N.Y. 125, 105 N.E. 92 (1914). The opinion, by Judge Benjamin Cardozo, is widely regarded as the foundational American statement of a patient's right to self-determination.

[2] *Salgo v. Leland Stanford Jr. University Board of Trustees*, 154 Cal. App. 2d 560 (1957), in which the term "informed consent" first appeared.

[3] *Canterbury v. Spence*, 464 F.2d 772 (D.C. Cir. 1972), which established the "reasonable patient" standard for how much a physician must disclose.

[4] Kutner M, Greenberg E, Jin Y, Paulsen C. *The Health Literacy of America's Adults: Results From the 2003 National Assessment of Adult Literacy* (NAAL). U.S. Department of Education, National Center for Education Statistics, 2006.

CHAPTER THREE
IS IT WORTH IT?

Frank is sixty-two, and his doctor has just offered him a pill. "This medication," she says, "cuts your risk of a heart attack by half."

By half. Frank doesn't need to hear another word. Cut a heart attack risk in half? Sign him up. Who would say no to that?

But hold on. Before Frank rolls up his sleeve, let's ask a question he didn't think to ask: *half of what?*

Suppose that out of 100 men just like Frank, 2 would have a heart attack over the next few years without the pill. With the pill, that drops to 1 out of 100. Is that "half"? Technically, yes — 1 is half of 2. The drug company can honestly say it cuts the risk by 50 percent. But look at what actually happened to those 100 men: 99 out of 100 were going to be fine either way. The pill helped exactly one of them.

"Cuts your risk in half" and "helps 1 man out of 100" describe the *exact same pill.* They just *feel* completely different. And that gap — between how a number sounds and what it actually means — is one of the most important things you will ever learn about your own health.

This chapter is about a single question that sits underneath every medical decision you'll ever make. Not "is this treatment good?" The real question is always: **is it worth it — for me?**

THE OLDEST TRICK IN THE NUMBERS

Every treatment is a trade-off. There is no such thing as a medicine that only helps and never harms, or a surgery with upside and no downside. So the whole game is weighing the good against the bad. And the very first thing that trips people up is the difference between two ways of describing a benefit.

The way that *sounds* impressive is called **relative risk** — "cuts your risk in half," "reduces deaths by 30 percent." The way that actually tells you what's happening is called **absolute risk** — "helps 1 person out of 100." Relative numbers almost always sound bigger. That's exactly why advertisements, headlines, and even some pamphlets love to use them.

Here's a real example that researchers have studied closely. Women are often told that getting a mammogram "reduces the risk of dying from breast cancer by about 25 percent." That sounds enormous. But when you look at the actual bodies, that 25 percent works out to roughly *one fewer death for every 1,000 women* who get screened over many years.[1] Both numbers are true. They describe the same thing. But one makes screening sound like a miracle and the other tells you its real size.

Now here's the part that should make all of us humble. When researchers checked how well women understood that real number, only about 6 out of 100 had it right. Many believed screening saved *80 or more* women out of every 1,000 — off by a factor of nearly a hundred.[1] These weren't foolish people. They had simply been handed the impressive-sounding version and never the honest one.

So here is your first and most powerful tool, and you can use it today, with any treatment, any test, any headline:

Ask: "How many out of 100?" (Or out of 1,000.) *How many people like me are helped if we all do this? How many are harmed? How many would have been fine anyway?* Real numbers, real people. If someone can only answer you in percentages and "reduces by half," politely ask them to translate it into how many actual people out of a hundred. Watch how often the picture changes.

HOW TO ACTUALLY WEIGH IT

Once you have the real numbers, weighing a decision comes down to three plain questions. Doctors do a version of this in their heads; there's no reason you can't do it out loud.

How likely? What are the odds this helps me, and what are the odds it hurts me? (In real numbers, not "half.")

How big a deal? Not all risks are equal. A 10 percent chance of a mild rash and a 10 percent chance of a stroke are both "10 percent," but they are not remotely the same decision. You have to weigh *how likely* against *how serious.*

How much does it matter to me? This is the question medicine often forgets, and it may be the most important one of all.

There's a phrase doctors use that's worth knowing, because it makes all of this concrete: the **number needed to treat.** It's just this — how many people have to take a treatment for one person to benefit? Sometimes the answer is 5, which is fantastic. Sometimes 100 people take a pill every day for years so that a single one of them avoids a heart attack. Is that worth it? Here's the honest truth: *that's not a medical question. It's a personal one.*

Let's put actual bodies to that. Say a medication has a number needed to treat of 100 for preventing a heart attack over five years. Line up 100 people who take that pill faithfully, every single morning, for five years, and here's what you get:

One of them avoids a heart attack they would otherwise have had. For that one person, this pill was enormous — possibly life-saving.

A handful get side effects: muscle aches, stomach trouble, something that nags at them daily.

All the rest — the large majority — swallow more than eighteen hundred pills apiece and get nothing whatsoever out of it, because they were never going to have a heart attack in those five years anyway.

Is that a good deal?

Reasonable people answer that differently, and both are thinking clearly. Someone with a strong family history and a real dread of heart disease may look at that and say *absolutely, and gladly.* Someone who already hates taking pills and gets side effects from everything may look at the identical numbers and say *not for me.*

There is no arithmetic that settles it. Because the last step of the calculation was never arithmetic at all. It's you.

WHY TWO PEOPLE SHOULD CHOOSE DIFFERENTLY

Remember the two patients from the very first chapter, saying yes and no to the same treatment? Risk and benefit is where that comes roaring back.

Picture the same medication offered to two different people. It carries a small risk — say, three chances in a hundred — of lasting nerve damage in the hands.

The first patient is a man named Ray, who drives a delivery route and has for twenty years. He hears "three in a hundred, nerve damage in the hands." He takes it seriously. He thinks about it overnight. And he decides he can live with those odds — ninety-seven out of a hundred come through this just fine. He starts the medication.

The second patient is a woman named Vivian. She is fifty-four, and she has been sitting at a piano since she was six years old. She teaches. She still performs. Her hands are not a body part to her; they are how she speaks, how she earns her living, and the reason a room full of people goes quiet on a Friday night.

For Vivian, "three chances in a hundred of nerve damage in the hands" is not the sentence Ray heard. The words are identical. The number is identical. But what is being put at risk is not remotely the same thing. She turns it down and asks what else there is.

Neither of them is being irrational. Neither of them is weighing it *wrong*. They are putting the very same number on two completely different scales.

This is the quiet truth at the center of this whole book: there is very rarely one "right" medical answer that fits everyone. The numbers are the same for all of us, but the weighing is personal, because *you* are part of the equation. What you love, what you fear, what kind of life you're trying to protect — all of it belongs on the scale. A good decision isn't just the one with the best statistics. It's the one that's best *for you.*

That means no one — not a doctor, not a pamphlet, not a well-meaning relative — can do the final weighing for you. They can hand you the numbers. Only you can supply the values.

YOU DON'T HAVE TO DO THIS ALONE

If all this sounds like a lot to carry, here's the good news: you don't have to carry it by yourself, and you don't have to become a statistician.

For many common decisions, there are tools called **decision aids** — simple guides, booklets, or short videos that lay out your options in plain numbers and walk you through what matters to you. And they work. Researchers gathered more than a hundred studies covering over twenty-five thousand people and found that when patients used these aids, they understood their choices better, judged the risks far more accurately, and took a more active role in their own care. Just as importantly, people who used them were *no more likely to regret their decisions* afterward — often less.[2] In other words, understanding the trade-off didn't make people anxious. It made them steadier.

So when you're facing a real decision, you can simply ask: "Is there a decision aid for this?" And you can always fall back on the questions from this chapter:

- What are the real numbers — how many out of 100 are helped, and how many harmed?
- How serious is each thing that could go wrong?
- What happens if I do nothing?
- And what matters most to *me* here?

WHAT FRANK ASKED

Frank asked.

He hadn't planned to. He was already reaching for his sleeve when something snagged in his mind, and what came out was: "Hang on — out of a hundred guys like me, how many does this actually help?"

His doctor didn't bristle. She pulled her chair around, which is what the good ones do, and gave him the real numbers. Without the pill, roughly 2 in 100 men his age with his numbers would have a heart attack over the next several years. With it, roughly 1. She told him about the side effects, too — muscle aches for some, nothing at all for most.

Frank sat with that a moment.

"So ninety-eight of us are fine either way."

"Ninety-eight of you," she agreed. "And I can't tell you which one you are. That's the honest answer."

Here's how it ended: Frank took the pill.

Same outcome he'd been about to choose anyway, four minutes earlier — but for entirely different reasons, and that difference is not small. He'd stopped being a man doing what he was told because a number sounded impressive. He'd become a man who understood the actual size of what he was buying: one chance in a hundred, at the price of a daily tablet and a possible ache. And he decided that trade was worth it to him.

He also walked out understanding what he was *not* buying. He didn't leave believing he was now safe. He left knowing he'd nudged the odds a little in his favor — which is what most of medicine actually does, most of the time.

That's not a smaller thing to know. It's a truer one.

THE GOOD NEWS

Frank's whole transformation took one sentence and about four minutes.

That single question changed him from someone having a decision handed to him into someone genuinely making one. He still ended up with the same pill in his hand — but now it was *his* choice, made with open eyes, weighed on *his* scale.

That's the real gift hiding inside risk and benefit. Numbers can feel cold and frightening, but they're really just a map. And once you know how to read a map, you're not lost anymore — you're the one deciding where to go. You don't need a medical degree. You just need to ask "how many out of 100?", to remember that how *serious* matters as much as how *likely*, and to put your own life honestly on the scale.

Do that, and you'll never again have to take anyone's word that something is "worth it." You'll be able to answer that question for yourself — which is exactly how it should be.

NOTES

[1] Gigerenzer G, Gaissmaier W, Kurz-Milcke E, Schwartz LM, Woloshin S. "Helping Doctors and Patients Make Sense of Health Statistics." *Psychological Science in the Public Interest.* 2007;8(2):53–96. The study of women's understanding of mammography's absolute benefit draws on Domenighetti G, et al. (2003), discussed therein.

[2] Stacey D, Lewis KB, Smith M, et al. "Decision Aids for People Facing Health Treatment or Screening Decisions." *Cochrane Database of Systematic Reviews.* 2024, Issue 1. Art. No.: CD001431. (Pooled findings across more than 100 studies and 25,000+ participants.)

CHAPTER FOUR
WHEN THE CHOICE ISN'T YOURS

Ellen watches her grown son, Danny, come apart over a matter of weeks. He stops sleeping. He stops eating. He starts saying things that don't connect to the world the rest of us live in — that the neighbors are sending him messages, that he has a mission no one else can understand. He is frightened, and he is frightening. And when Ellen begs him to see a doctor, he looks at her like she's the enemy and slams the door.

So Ellen does what any of us would do. She calls for help. And she runs straight into a wall she never knew existed. Danny is an adult. He has not committed a crime. And in America, you cannot simply force a competent adult into treatment because you love them and you're afraid for them.

Ellen is furious. *He's clearly not okay — why won't anyone help me help him?*

It's one of the most agonizing walls a family can hit. And here is the strange, important truth this chapter is about: that wall is there on purpose. It is there to protect Danny. It is there, in a quieter way, to protect *you.* And understanding why is one of the most important things a person can learn about the line between care and control.

THE MOST SERIOUS POWER A SOCIETY HAS

Think about what we're actually talking about. Forcing someone into treatment means taking away their freedom — locking a door, holding a person somewhere they don't want to be — even though they've broken no law. That is one of the gravest powers any society can hand to anyone. And history has taught us, in the hardest way, what happens when that power has no limits.

For much of the last century, it barely did. People could be committed to psychiatric hospitals on the say-so of a relative and a doctor, and simply... stay there. For years. Sometimes for life.

Consider a man named Kenneth Donaldson. In 1957, he was committed to a Florida state hospital. He wasn't dangerous. He wasn't getting meaningful treatment. He kept asking to leave, and people on the outside offered to help him. He was held anyway — for nearly *fifteen years.* His case went all the way to the U.S. Supreme Court, and in 1975 the Court said something that changed everything: a state cannot lock away a person who is not dangerous and who could live safely in freedom, on their own or with the help of willing family and friends.[1]

Read that again, because it's the hinge everything else swings on. Being ill is not enough. Being strange, or frightening to your family, or making choices other people hate — none of that is enough. In a free country, the mere fact that you need help does not give anyone the right to force it on you.

Which is exactly why Ellen hit that wall. The wall is the lesson of Kenneth Donaldson's fifteen years.

SO WHEN *CAN* THE CHOICE BE TAKEN AWAY?

If illness alone isn't enough, what is? Society draws the line at one word: **danger.**

But "danger" comes in more than one form, and the law recognizes each of them. The most obvious is danger to *other people* — the same basic reason we let the state step in against any threat to public safety. The second is immediate danger to *oneself* — a person in the grip of a crisis who is at real risk of self-harm. And there is a third form, quieter and easy to miss, but every bit as real: when severe illness leaves a person unable to keep *themselves* alive at all. The law has a name for that last one — being *gravely disabled* — and because it's where families most often feel the system has abandoned them, it's worth understanding on its own.

And even then, the bar is deliberately high. It isn't enough to believe someone is ill and might be in danger. In a case called *Addington v. Texas,* the Supreme Court ruled that before the state can commit someone, it has to prove both mental illness *and* dangerousness by what the law calls **"clear and convincing evidence."**[2] That's a specific, meaningful standard. It's much stronger than a coin-flip "more likely than not." It's not quite as absolute as the "beyond a reasonable doubt" we demand to send someone to prison. It sits deliberately in between — high enough to guard against mistakes and misuse, because someone's freedom is on the line, but not so high that we can never protect a person in genuine danger.

In plain terms: the law is trying to make it *hard,* but not *impossible,* to take away a person's choice. That difficulty is not a bug. It's the whole design.

THE SLOW DANGER: BEING "GRAVELY DISABLED"

Not every emergency looks like a threat. Sometimes the danger is simply that a person has become so ill that they can no longer take care of themselves at all.

Consider a man named Marcus. He's thirty-four, warm and funny when he's well, and for three weeks now he has been climbing — talking faster than anyone can follow, awake for days at a stretch, certain he has been chosen for something enormous. He hasn't threatened a soul. He is, if anything, joyful.

But he hasn't eaten a real meal in a week, because eating feels like a waste of precious time. He has given away his car and most of his savings to strangers. He has walked into traffic twice — not to harm himself, but because he simply didn't register the cars. And when his sister begs him to see a doctor, he laughs and tells her she doesn't understand: he has never felt better in his life.

That last part is the cruelest detail, and it's the one families find hardest to explain to anyone who hasn't seen it. Marcus isn't lying. He genuinely feels wonderful. The illness has taken away the very faculty he would need in order to notice that he's in danger.

He is not a threat to anyone. He has simply stopped sleeping, stopped eating, stopped recognizing that the body he lives in has needs at all. He can no longer organize the simple, life-sustaining acts — food, shelter, warmth, medicine — that the rest of us manage without thinking. He is, quietly and dangerously, running out of the ability to keep himself alive.

The law calls this being **gravely disabled:** unable, because of a mental illness, to provide for your own basic needs — food, clothing, shelter, and in many places medical care and personal safety. It's danger on a slower fuse. Nothing terrible has to happen today. But left alone, a person in that state is a kind of ticking clock, and everyone who loves them can hear it even when the person themselves cannot. Nearly every state recognizes grave disability as a reason a person's choice can be set aside — precisely because "just wait until they're actually harmed" is a cruel, and sometimes deadly, thing to ask of a family.[3]

And notice the safeguard built right into it — the very same one from Kenneth Donaldson's case. Illness alone is never enough. The question is never whether a person is sick, or eccentric, or living in a way we wouldn't choose. It's whether they can actually meet their own basic needs to survive. If they can do that safely with the help of a willing family member or friend, then in the eyes of the law they generally are *not* gravely disabled. The standard reaches only genuine inability to survive — never unusual lives, unpopular choices, or people others simply find hard to understand.

WHAT IT ACTUALLY LOOKS LIKE

In a true emergency — someone in immediate danger of harming themselves or another person, or so gravely ill they can no longer keep themselves alive — the first step is usually a short **emergency hold.** A doctor or sometimes an officer can have the person taken to a hospital and kept there, typically for up to about 72 hours, purely so trained people can evaluate what's happening. (The exact rules and time limits vary from state to state, which is why it's worth knowing your own state's law.) An emergency hold is a pause, not a sentence. It exists to buy time and safety, nothing more.

To hold someone longer than that takes far more: a court, a hearing, a judge, evidence, and — crucially — the person's right to be released the moment they are no longer dangerous. There are lawyers. There are reviews. And running through all of it is a principle worth remembering, because you can hold anyone to it: the **least restrictive option.** The system is required to reach for the gentlest tool that will keep the person safe, not the heaviest one. If someone can be safe at home with support, they shouldn't be in a locked ward.

BEING ORDERED TO GET TREATMENT — WHILE LIVING YOUR LIFE

There's also a middle path that surprises people. Sometimes a court doesn't send a person to a hospital at all. Instead, it orders them to keep up with treatment — appointments, medication, check-ins — while continuing to live at home, in their own community.

New York's version is called **Kendra's Law,** named for Kendra Webdale, a young woman who died in 1999 after being pushed in front of a subway train by a man with untreated serious mental illness. Under this kind of order — versions of which now exist in most states — a judge can require someone with a history of crisis and repeated hospitalizations to stick with a treatment plan.[4] State evaluations and independent researchers have linked these programs to fewer hospitalizations, arrests, and episodes of homelessness among the people under them.

And yet — in the spirit of this whole book, which never pretends the hard questions are easy — thoughtful people genuinely disagree about this. Supporters see a compassionate way to keep vulnerable people stable and out of hospitals and jails. Civil-liberties advocates worry about the state ordering treatment for people who aren't actually dangerous, and about where that power might drift. Both sides are arguing, in good faith, over the same two precious things: keeping people safe, and keeping people free. That tension never fully resolves. It's the price of taking both values seriously.

THE HUMAN HEART OF IT

Step back into the hospital room for a moment, and see it from the inside. To a person in crisis, being held can feel like the ultimate betrayal — like being punished for being sick, locked up by the very people who claim to care. That feeling is real, and it deserves respect, not dismissal. Anyone working in this field who has forgotten how terrifying it is to lose your freedom has lost something they needed to keep.

But here is the other half of the truth, and it matters just as much. At its best, this is not a prison. It's a safety net stretched beneath someone during the worst storm of their life — a way to keep them alive and whole until the storm passes. And it usually does pass. Most people stabilize. Most people go home. The entire point of every rule in this chapter — the proof standards, the judges, the time limits, the "least restrictive option," the right to walk out the moment the danger lifts — is to make sure the power is used as *care,* and only for as long as care requires.

WHAT HAPPENED TO DANNY

Ellen's story didn't end at that closed door.

Over the following weeks, Danny got worse. He stopped eating. He stopped sleeping almost entirely. He stopped opening his mail, and then he stopped opening his door. When Ellen finally let herself into his apartment, she found a man who had lost fifteen pounds in a month and who looked at her without quite recognizing her.

This time, when she called for help, the answer was different — not because anyone had changed their mind about Danny's rights, but because *Danny had changed.* He was no longer simply a frightened adult refusing care. He had crossed into that other territory: a person who could no longer meet his own basic needs to survive.

Danny was taken to a hospital on an emergency hold. Ellen has said since that it was the worst day of her life and the day she saved her son's life, and that both of those things are true at once.

He was furious with her. For three days he wouldn't speak to her at all, and when he finally did, he told her she had betrayed him. She sat in the parking lot afterward and wondered whether she had.

He stabilized in about two weeks. He was home in three. There was no long confinement, no drawn-out court battle, no institution — the hold did precisely what it was designed to do: keep him alive and safe for the short stretch of time it took for treatment to work and for his own judgment to find its way back to him.

It was nearly a year before Danny brought it up himself. They were in her kitchen. He said, quietly, that he didn't remember most of that month — but that he remembered being *certain,* absolutely certain, that nothing was wrong with him.

And then he thanked her.

Not every story goes this way. Some are harder, some are longer, and some don't resolve at all. But Danny's is worth telling because it is the ordinary outcome — the one that never makes the news. A person in crisis, held briefly and lawfully, treated, and handed back his own life with his freedom intact.

That is the system working. Not as a cage. As a bridge.

WHAT THIS MEANS FOR YOU

If you ever stand where Ellen stood — frightened for someone you love, or facing this yourself — you are not helpless, and you are not without rights. You can ask the questions that keep the system honest:

Why exactly is this person being held? What's the actual evidence of danger?

What are their rights, and when will a court review this?

What's the least restrictive option that would keep them safe?

When and how does this end?

Knowing those questions doesn't just make you informed. It makes you a guardian of the safeguards — for your loved one, and for the stranger down the hall who has no one asking on their behalf.

THE GOOD NEWS

This is the heaviest power in all of medicine: the power to say, for a little while, that the choice is not yours. It would be easy for a society to use that power carelessly, or cruelly, or not at all. Ours tries to do something harder and better — to hold two precious things in the same hand at once. To keep people safe *and* to keep people free. To step in when someone truly cannot protect themselves, and to step back the instant they can.

We don't always get the balance right. But the fact that we surround this power with judges and evidence and time limits and the promise of freedom returned — that is not weakness. It is a society insisting that even its most frightened, most unwell members are still people, still owed their dignity, still owed their way home.

And that way home is the whole point. Because the goal, always, is not to hold someone. It's to help them through the storm, and then hand their life gently back — their freedom, their choices, their future — right where it belongs, in their own hands.

NOTES

[1] *O'Connor v. Donaldson*, 422 U.S. 563 (1975). The Court held that a state cannot constitutionally confine a non-dangerous individual who is capable of surviving safely in freedom by themselves or with the help of willing family or friends.

[2] *Addington v. Texas*, 441 U.S. 418 (1979). The Court held that due process requires proof by "clear and convincing evidence" — a standard between the

ordinary civil "preponderance of the evidence" and the criminal "beyond a reasonable doubt" — before an individual may be involuntarily committed.

[3] The "gravely disabled" standard was codified in California's Lanterman-Petris-Short Act (1967) and was subsequently adopted by most states. It is typically defined as being unable, as a result of mental illness, to provide for one's basic personal needs such as food, clothing, and shelter (see, e.g., Cal. Welf. & Inst. Code § 5008(h)). As of 2020, only a small number of U.S. jurisdictions lacked a grave-disability basis for civil commitment. Precise definitions, added criteria (such as medical care or personal safety), and procedures vary by state.

[4] Kendra's Law, New York Mental Hygiene Law § 9.60 (enacted 1999), the state's Assisted Outpatient Treatment (AOT) statute. Comparable involuntary-outpatient-treatment laws exist in most U.S. states. Outcome findings are drawn from evaluations by the New York State Office of Mental Health and independent researchers; exact criteria, procedures, and time limits vary by state.

CHAPTER FIVE
WHOSE SAY IS IT?

Eli is six. He sits on the exam table swinging his legs, spots the nurse coming with the needle, and says "No." He means it with his whole body — arms crossed, chin tucked, tears already starting. It is the most sincere "no" a human being can produce.

Nora is sixteen. She sits on that same table a few years later, in that same clinic. She's been offered a treatment. She has thought about it, read about it, asked two people she trusts, and slept on it. And she says "No" too — calm, clear, and full of reasons she can explain to you one by one.

Same word. Same table. But almost everyone senses right away that these two "no"s don't carry the same weight. We would hold Eli's hand, count to three, and give him the shot anyway — and we'd be right to. Nora's "no" stops us cold. It makes us sit down and listen.

Why?

That question — *whose say is it?* — turns out to be one of the trickiest in all of medicine, because the answer isn't a number. It's a dial that slowly turns as a child grows up. A young person is never quite a little adult who can decide everything. But they are never property, either. Somewhere in between is a moving line, and this chapter is about how we find it, kindly and fairly, at every age.

START WITH A SIMPLE TRUTH: KIDS GET A VOICE, EVEN WHEN THEY DON'T GET THE VOTE

For a young child, parents are the decision-makers. That's not the law being harsh; it's the law being realistic. Eli can't weigh a treatment's risks against its benefits, so someone who loves him has to do it for him, guided by a single question: what's genuinely best for this child?

But — and this matters more than most people realize — "the parents decide" does not mean "the child is ignored." Doctors have a name for the difference. The parents give *permission.* The child, whenever they're old enough to understand anything at all, is asked for their **assent** — their agreement, in their own small way. The American Academy of Pediatrics has urged for decades that children be brought into their own care as much as their age allows: told what's about to happen, in words they can grasp, and asked how they feel about it.[1]

Why bother, if the parents have the final say anyway? Because a child who is told the truth and treated as a person — even a very young one — learns that medicine is something done *with* them, not *to* them. That lesson shapes how they'll walk into a doctor's office for the rest of their life. Assent isn't a legal technicality. It's the beginning of respect.

PARENTS HAVE POWER — BUT NOT UNLIMITED POWER

Here's something that surprises people: a parent's authority over a child's medical care, real as it is, has limits. And the limit is the child's own welfare.

Most of the time, parents and the child's best interest point in exactly the same direction — that's why we trust parents in the first place. But every so often, they don't. The hardest example is a parent who, out of sincere religious conviction, refuses a treatment their child needs to survive. What happens then?

The answer came from the Supreme Court back in 1944, in a case called *Prince v. Massachusetts,* and its logic has shaped the law ever since. The Court's memorable idea was this: adults are free to make sacrifices — even to become martyrs — for their own beliefs. But they are *not* free to make that same sacrifice of their child, who hasn't yet reached the age to choose such a thing for themselves.[2] In plain terms: you can take a grave risk with your own life for your faith. You cannot take it with your child's.

So when a child's life is genuinely on the line, the state can step in and authorize treatment over a parent's objection. This isn't the government barging into family life for sport — courts are deeply reluctant, and it happens only in serious cases. The reasoning is quietly beautiful: protecting the child's life today preserves their chance to grow up and one day make these profound choices — about faith, about their own body — for themselves. Parental love is the rule. The child's right to reach adulthood is the limit.

THE TEEN ZONE: WHERE THE DIAL TURNS FAST

Between Eli and the young adult he will become lies the most interesting stretch of all — the teenage years, when that dial starts turning in earnest.

Two things happen here. First, the law in many places recognizes what's called the **mature minor doctrine:** a teenager who is genuinely able to understand a particular decision may, in some situations, be allowed to make it, even without a parent's sign-off. Maturity, not just age, starts to count.

Second — and this is the part most families never learn until they need it — nearly every state has passed specific laws letting minors consent, on their own and confidentially, to certain kinds of sensitive care. All fifty states let a minor get tested and treated for sexually transmitted infections without a parent's permission. Many states let teens, often from around age twelve, consent on their own to mental health counseling, to treatment for drug or alcohol problems, and to contraception.[3]

Now, why on earth would the law cut parents out of decisions like these? It sounds backwards. But there's a hard, compassionate logic behind it, and it's worth understanding. Lawmakers looked at reality and saw a painful truth: if a frightened teenager has to tell a parent before they can get help, a great many of them simply *won't get help at all.* They'll let the infection go untreated. They'll suffer the depression in silence. They'll hide the addiction until it's much worse. So the law made a deliberate bet — that a teen who can quietly get care is far better off than a teen who gets none. It isn't a vote against parents. It's a safety net for the kids who, in a crisis, feel they can't reach their parents.

Here's what that bet looks like in a real life.

A girl — call her Maya — is fifteen. Somewhere in the middle of her sophomore year, things get dark. She stops sleeping well. She stops seeing her friends. She starts believing she's a burden to everyone around her, which is the kind of thought that feeds on itself in the quiet.

She doesn't tell her parents. Not because they're cruel — they aren't, and they love her — but because she is fifteen and convinced that telling them would devastate them, or disappoint them, or turn into A Whole Thing she doesn't have the strength for right now. So she says nothing. For months.

What she does do, eventually, is walk into the school counselor's office, and then into a clinic — because someone happened to mention that she could go on her own. She gets evaluated. She starts seeing a therapist. It helps. Not overnight, but it helps.

A few weeks later, with her therapist sitting beside her, she tells her mother.

Her mother's reaction is the one nearly every parent has, and it arrives in two waves. The first is relief so enormous it nearly takes her legs out from under her. The second, right behind it, is harder: *Why didn't she come to me? Why was I the last to know?*

That second feeling is real, and it deserves to be honored rather than argued with. It isn't selfish. It's the particular grief of a parent who would have moved mountains and never got the chance.

But sit with the alternative for a moment. If Maya had needed permission to walk through that clinic door, she would not have walked through it. Not that month. Possibly not that year. The choice was never *"her parents find out now"* versus *"her parents find out later."* It was *"she gets help"* versus *"she doesn't."*

These laws exist for the months in between — that stretch when a kid genuinely cannot bring themselves to tell you, and still needs someone. They're not a wall between you and your child.

They're a bridge your child can use to get back to you.

WHEN THE TEEN AND THE PARENT DISAGREE

Of course, this is exactly where things get emotionally raw. A parent who discovers their child sought care without them can feel shut out, even betrayed — *I'm their mother; how could I not be told?* And a teenager fighting for a say can feel controlled, not cared for. Both feelings are real. Both usually come from the same place: love, tangled up with fear.

There are genuine gray areas here that thoughtful people wrestle with — how much confidentiality a struggling teen should have, when a parent truly needs to be brought in, how to handle the hardest subjects. This book won't pretend those questions have easy answers. They don't. They sit right on the line between a young person's growing independence and a parent's enduring responsibility, and that line is tender for a reason.

One very practical thing worth knowing, because it trips up families constantly: even when the law lets a teen get confidential care, confidentiality can quietly break at the most ordinary moment — when the insurance bill or an "explanation of benefits" arrives in a parent's mailbox. The law and the paperwork don't always agree. If confidential care matters in your family's situation, it's worth asking the clinic directly how billing is handled.

WHAT THIS MEANS FOR YOU

If you're a **parent,** here's the reframe that helps most: the goal was never to win a power struggle. It's to raise a young person who can one day make good decisions without you in the room — because someday you won't be. Every time you explain instead of just deciding, every time you let their voice grow a little, you're not losing authority. You're doing the actual job.

If you're a **young person,** know that you have more of a voice, and often more rights, than you might think — especially around sensitive care. You're allowed to ask, "Is this confidential? Who will know?" You're allowed to be part of the conversation about your own body.

And for anyone in the room, the questions stay simple:

Is this child being included as much as their age allows?

What is truly in this child's best interest — not just the adults' comfort?

For a teen: what can they decide for themselves here, and what stays private?

WHAT HAPPENED TO ELI AND NORA

Eli got his shot.

He cried, and then he had a sticker on his shirt, and by the parking lot he'd mostly forgotten about it. That was the right call, and nobody should agonize over it.

But here's what his pediatrician did that mattered more than the shot itself. Before the needle came out, she crouched down to his eye level and told him what was about to happen, in words a six-year-old actually owns: that it would pinch, that it would be over fast, that he could squeeze his mom's hand as hard as he wanted, and that it was okay to cry.

He still said no. She still gave it to him. But he wasn't ambushed.

Six years later, at twelve, Eli is the one asking the doctor what the medicine does. At fifteen, he's the one describing his own symptoms while his mother sits in the corner biting her tongue — which is one of the harder things a parent is ever asked to do. At eighteen, he goes in alone, and he's ready.

Nobody handed him that at eighteen. It got built, one visit at a time, out of a hundred small moments where an adult explained instead of simply deciding.

And Nora? Nora's "no" got taken seriously.

Her doctor asked what worried her — and it turned out her reasons were good ones. She'd read about a side effect that would have wrecked something that mattered a great deal to her, and nobody had thought to bring it up. They found a different approach together.

She might have been wrong. Teenagers sometimes are, and so is everyone else. But she was *heard.* And what she learned in that room is the thing this entire chapter is about: that her voice counts in the place where decisions about her own body get made.

She will carry that into every exam room she ever walks into for the rest of her life.

THE GOOD NEWS

Growing up is, in a way, this exact process, stretched over eighteen years: the slow, loving handing-over of the keys to your own life. It doesn't happen with a bang on a single birthday. It happens gradually — a little more voice, a little more trust, a little more responsibility, year after year.

Good medicine mirrors good parenting here, and that's the hopeful part. Neither one flips a switch at eighteen and says, "Now you're on your own." Both do something gentler and wiser: they turn the dial a notch at a time, walking beside the child as their voice grows louder and their judgment grows surer, until one day the young person is ready to hold their own life fully in their own hands.

That dial turning isn't a threat to anyone's authority. It's the whole point of raising a human being. It means the frightened six-year-old on that exam table — Eli, with his arms crossed and his chin tucked — is becoming a person — one who will, in time, be able to sit on that table alone, weigh a hard choice, and decide, with confidence, what's right for the one life that is truly theirs.

And helping a child become that person may be the most important thing any of us ever does.

NOTES

[1] American Academy of Pediatrics, Committee on Bioethics. "Informed Consent in Decision-Making in Pediatric Practice." *Pediatrics.* 2016;138(2):e20161484 (reaffirmed 2023); building on the Committee's earlier statement, "Informed Consent, Parental Permission, and Assent in Pediatric Practice," *Pediatrics.* 1995;95(2):314–317.

[2] *Prince v. Massachusetts*, 321 U.S. 158 (1944). The Court held that parental authority and religious freedom are not without limits where a child's welfare is at stake, and that the state may act to protect a child even over a parent's sincere objection.

[3] Guttmacher Institute, "Minors and the Right to Consent to Health Care," and related state-law analyses. All 50 states and the District of Columbia allow minors to consent to STI testing and treatment; many additionally allow minors to consent to contraceptive services, outpatient mental health care, and substance-use treatment. Specific ages, services, and confidentiality rules vary by state and change over time.

CHAPTER SIX
KNOWING WHEN TO LET GO

Grace is standing in a hospital hallway at the worst moment of her life. Her father, Sam, is dying — his body worn out after a long illness, his good days behind him. A doctor comes out, kind and tired, and asks the question that families dread most:

"Do you want us to do everything we can?"

And Grace hears herself say it instantly, the way almost anyone would: "Yes. Of course. Do everything."

Because what else could love possibly say? To answer anything less feels like giving up on her father, like failing him at the one moment he needs her most.

But here is the gentlest, hardest truth in this entire book, and it's the reason this chapter exists: sometimes "do everything" is not the most loving answer. Sometimes the bravest, kindest, most loving thing a family can do is to stop trying to win an unwinnable fight — and instead make the time that's left as peaceful, as comfortable, and as full of love as it can possibly be.

That's not giving up. As we'll see, it's often the truest form of caring there is.

THE QUESTION BEHIND THE QUESTION

When a doctor asks, "Do you want us to do everything?", the word *everything* hides a trap. It can mean two completely different things.

It can mean every machine, every tube, every last aggressive intervention — chest compressions that crack ribs, a breathing machine, more time in an ICU. Or it can mean everything to keep someone comfortable, everything to ease their pain, everything to let them spend their final days at home, awake, surrounded by the people they love.

Both are "everything." They just point in opposite directions. So the real question — the one worth asking out loud — was never simply "do everything?" It's this: *What kind of time does my father have left, and what would make that time good?*

Once you ask it that way, the whole conversation changes.

TWO MYTHS WE NEED TO SET DOWN

Most of us walk into that hallway carrying two beliefs that feel obviously true but that the evidence gently overturns.

The first myth: more treatment always means more life. It seems like common sense. Fight harder, live longer. But consider what researchers found in a landmark study of patients with a very serious lung cancer. One group got the usual aggressive cancer treatment. The other got that same treatment *plus* palliative care — comfort-focused care aimed at easing symptoms and protecting quality of life from the start. The comfort-care group felt better. They were less depressed. They chose less aggressive treatment near the end. And here is the part that stunned even the doctors: *they lived longer* — a median of about 11.6 months, compared with 8.9 months for the group getting aggressive treatment alone.[1]

Read that again. The people who focused on comfort didn't die sooner for it. They lived *longer* — and better. As one of the study's doctors put it, the biggest misconception about this kind of care is the belief that it means treatment has failed, that it means giving up. It doesn't. Sometimes tending to comfort is exactly what helps a person live.

The second myth: doing everything is always the loving choice. Here the evidence is even more sobering, and more important. In another major study, researchers followed people dying of cancer and then followed the families they left behind. Patients who received very aggressive medical care in their final days had *worse* quality of life at the end. And their loved ones paid a price too: caregivers of patients who died in that aggressive way were markedly more likely to develop major depression in their grief. Meanwhile, patients who received hospice care had better quality of life in their final days.[2]

Sit with what that means. How a person dies doesn't end with them. It echoes — for years — in the hearts of everyone who loved them. A peaceful death can be a final gift to a family. A harrowing one can become a wound that grief never quite closes. "Doing everything," in the aggressive sense, can hurt not only the person we're trying to save but the people we'll go on living beside.

WHAT HOSPICE AND PALLIATIVE CARE ACTUALLY ARE

Because these words scare people, let's say plainly what they mean.

Palliative care is comfort care — treatment aimed at easing pain and symptoms and protecting your quality of life. It is *not* only for the dying. You can receive it at any stage of a serious illness, right alongside treatments meant to cure or control the disease. It's not either-or.

Hospice is comfort care for when a cure is no longer the goal — when the focus shifts from fighting the illness to making whatever time remains as full, as comfortable, and as peaceful as possible. Hospice is not a place you're sent to die. It's a kind of care, often given right at home, built around a simple idea: that the end of a life still deserves tenderness, dignity, and as many good moments as we can gather.

Here's the reframe that helps most: choosing comfort care is not choosing to die. It's choosing *how to live* the time you have left. It's a decision about living, right up to the very end.

"SHOULD WE TREAT, OR LET NATURE TAKE ITS COURSE?"

This brings us to the question families agonize over: when is it right to stop?

The honest answer, in the spirit of this whole book, is that there's no formula that fits everyone — because it depends on what you're treating *for.* A treatment that buys three more months, but spends them in a hospital, sedated and in pain, is a very different thing from two good months at home, awake, holding your grandchildren. Neither choice is "right" for everybody. The right one depends on the person, their values, and what a good day looks like *to them.*

What's crucial to know — because so many families don't — is that saying "enough" is entirely allowed. A competent adult has a long-recognized legal and moral right to refuse or to stop medical treatment, even treatment that is keeping them alive. Our courts affirmed this decades ago.[3] And families speaking for a loved one who can no longer speak share in that right.

And here's something important to be at peace with: choosing to stop treatment, or to not start it, is *not* the same as causing death. When we let an illness run its natural course, it is the illness — not the choice, not the family — that brings the end. Letting nature take its course is not abandoning someone. For countless families, it is the final, loving act of accepting what medicine cannot change, and choosing to spend the remaining time on love instead of on machines.

A WORD ON "DEATH WITH DIGNITY"

You may hear the phrase "death with dignity," and it's worth understanding, because it means two related but different things.

Broadly, it means dying comfortably and on your own terms — free of needless pain, surrounded by the people and things you love. That kind of dignified death is something hospice and palliative care can offer to nearly everyone, and it's what most people mean when they use the phrase.

More specifically, "medical aid in dying" refers to laws — in a minority of U.S. states and the District of Columbia, with the first enacted in Oregon and taking effect in 1997 — that allow a terminally ill, mentally capable adult to request medication to bring about a peaceful death on their own terms.[4] These laws carry strict safeguards, and they are genuinely, deeply debated. Some see them as the ultimate act of personal freedom and mercy. Others, on moral or religious grounds, believe hastening death is never the right path, and worry about the pressures such laws might place on the vulnerable. Both views are held sincerely, by thoughtful people, and this book won't tell you which to hold. It's worth knowing, though, that even where these laws exist, most people who use them are also receiving hospice care — a reminder that this is one option along a wide spectrum of end-of-life choices, not a substitute for comfort and love.

WHAT THIS MEANS FOR YOU

If you ever stand where Grace stood, you are not helpless, and you are allowed to slow the moment down and ask better questions:

What are we actually hoping this treatment will accomplish?

How much time might it add — and what *kind* of time? At home or in a hospital? Awake or sedated? In comfort or in pain?

What would a genuinely good day look like for my loved one now?

Is comfort care — palliative care or hospice — available to us?

And above all: what would *they* want, if they could tell us right now?

That last question is the compass. When you can't decide what *you* want for them, ask what *they* would want for themselves. It turns an impossible choice into an act of love: not choosing to lose them, but choosing to honor them.

WHAT GRACE CHOSE

Grace didn't answer the doctor that night. She asked him something instead.

"What kind of time would he actually have? If we do everything — what do the next few weeks look like for him?"

The doctor, who had been waiting for someone to ask, told her the truth. More aggressive treatment might buy some time, most of it spent in a hospital, much of it sedated, with a real possibility that Sam would never say another clear sentence to her.

Or they could take him home.

They took him home.

Sam lived nineteen more days. Hospice set up a bed in the front room by the window he liked, and taught Grace how to manage his medication so that he was comfortable and still awake. A nurse came every day. Someone was on the phone whenever they needed one at 3 a.m., and twice they did.

Those nineteen days were not easy, and they were not beautiful in the way people sometimes pretend. He was tired. There were hard nights. Grace was exhausted in a way she hadn't known was possible.

But her brother flew in, and the three of them watched a ball game together. Sam told a story about his own father that Grace had never heard before — and she has it now, and she'll have it for the rest of her life. The grandchildren came and went and weren't frightened, because there were no machines to be frightened of. He said something to an old friend that he'd been carrying for forty years, and was forgiven, and slept better afterward.

He died in that front room, early in the morning, holding his daughter's hand.

Grace will tell you she has grieved him hard. She will also tell you that she has never once lain awake wondering whether she failed him.

That second part is not a small thing. That is very nearly everything.

THE GOOD NEWS

We tend to think of letting go as failure — as the moment we stopped fighting, gave up, lost. But that isn't what it is at all.

Letting go, done with love, is not the opposite of caring. It is one of its highest forms. It takes more courage to stop an exhausting, futile fight and sit quietly at a bedside than it does to demand one more machine. It asks more of us to trade the illusion of control for the reality of presence

— to hold a hand instead of watching a monitor, to fill a room with old stories and quiet laughter instead of alarms.

A death that is peaceful, comfortable, free of needless pain, and surrounded by love is not a defeat. It may be one of the last and greatest gifts we ever give the people we love — and one of the last they give us. And knowing that such a death is possible, that we can choose comfort and presence and peace, means none of us has to face the end as a terrifying loss of control.

It can be, instead, a final chapter written with tenderness. Not a fight lost — but a life honored, all the way to its close.

And there is real peace in knowing that when the time comes, we get to choose how that story ends.

NOTES

[1] Temel JS, Greer JA, Muzikansky A, et al. "Early Palliative Care for Patients with Metastatic Non–Small-Cell Lung Cancer." *New England Journal of Medicine.* 2010;363(8):733–742. Patients receiving early palliative care alongside standard treatment reported better quality of life and mood, received less aggressive end-of-life care, and had longer median survival (11.6 vs. 8.9 months).

[2] Wright AA, Zhang B, Ray A, et al. "Associations Between End-of-Life Discussions, Patient Mental Health, Medical Care Near Death, and Caregiver Bereavement Adjustment." *JAMA.* 2008;300(14):1665–1673. Aggressive care near death was associated with worse patient quality of life and a higher risk of major depression among bereaved caregivers; hospice care was associated with better patient quality of life.

[3] *Cruzan v. Director, Missouri Department of Health*, 497 U.S. 261 (1990), in which the U.S. Supreme Court recognized that a competent person has a

constitutionally protected liberty interest in refusing unwanted life-sustaining medical treatment.

[4] Oregon's Death with Dignity Act took effect in 1997, the first such law in the United States. Medical aid in dying is now authorized in a minority of U.S. jurisdictions under strict eligibility and procedural safeguards; the U.S. Supreme Court in *Washington v. Glucksberg* (1997) held there is no constitutional right to it, leaving the matter to individual states. The number of states continues to change, so readers should check current law where they live.

CHAPTER SEVEN

WHEN SOMEONE ELSE HAS TO DECIDE

Tom is fifty-eight, healthy on Tuesday, and by Wednesday afternoon he's in a hospital bed after a sudden stroke, unable to speak or to tell anyone what he wants. In the waiting room sit the people who love him most: his wife, and his two grown children. A doctor lays out a decision that has to be made about his care, and turns to them.

And that's when the second crisis begins — the quiet one. Because Tom's wife leans one way, his son leans another, and his daughter says, through tears, the thing that hangs over every family in this situation: "I don't even know what Dad would *want.*»

Three people who all love the same man, all trying to do right by him, and no map for how. This chapter is about that moment — when a person can no longer decide for themselves, and someone else has to step in. And it turns out there are two separate questions hiding inside it, each with an answer worth knowing before you ever need it: *How* should the decision be made? And *who* gets to make it?

HOW: DECIDING THE WAY *THEY* WOULD

When you're deciding for someone who can't decide for themselves, ethics gives you a clear order of priorities — and it's built, from top to bottom, around one idea: *it's still their life, so keep it as much their decision as possible.*

First, look for their own instructions. If the person wrote down what they wanted — in a living will or similar document — that comes first. It's the closest thing to hearing their own voice, and we'll spend the whole final chapter on how to leave that gift.

If there's no written instruction, use what's called substituted judgment. This is a beautiful idea, and a demanding one. It asks you to step into the person's shoes and choose *not what you would want, but what they would have wanted* — using everything you know about their values, their beliefs, the offhand comments they made watching the news, the way they lived. The question is never "What do I want for Tom?" It's "What would *Tom* choose, if he could?"

And only if you truly cannot know — because they never told you, or never could — do you fall back to the best-interest standard: simply choosing what would be genuinely good for them, the way a caring, reasonable person would.[1] This is the standard we use for someone who has never been able to make such decisions at all.

Notice the whole ladder leans one direction: toward the person's own voice, and away from ours. That's the point.

THE HUMBLING TRUTH ABOUT GUESSING

Here's something that should make every family gentle with itself: even people who love someone deeply are not very good at guessing what that person would want. When researchers studied how accurately family members predicted their loved ones' medical wishes, they found surrogates guessed correctly only about two-thirds of the time — not much better than a coin flip on the genuinely hard calls.[2]

Two-thirds. From spouses. From children. Not because they didn't love the person — but because we almost never actually *ask* each other these questions until it's too late.

And there's a subtler trap, one every honest family should watch for. In the fog of fear and grief, it's terribly easy to slide from "what would *he* want" into "what can *I* not bear to lose" — to reach for one more day for our own sake and quietly tell ourselves it's for theirs. That slide is human and forgivable. But the discipline of substituted judgment is to catch it: to keep asking about *them,* not us. The most loving thing Tom's family can do is set down their own longing long enough to ask, honestly, what Tom himself would choose. Loving someone that way — choosing for them as *they* would, even when it costs you — may be one of the hardest and truest forms of love there is.

WHO: THE TWO VERY DIFFERENT PATHS

Now the second question: who has the actual authority to make the call? There are two paths to that authority, and they could hardly be more different.

The first path is a power of attorney — specifically, a healthcare power of attorney, sometimes called a healthcare proxy or agent. This is something *you* set up, in advance, while you're well and thinking clearly. You simply name the person you trust to speak for you if you ever can't. There's no court, no judge, no delay. And your agent is bound to follow *your* wishes. A power of attorney is, at heart, an act of self-determination: you choosing, ahead of time, who will carry your voice.[3]

The second path is guardianship (called conservatorship in some places). This is what happens when you *didn't* name anyone — or the person you named can't serve, or you were never able to make such choices in the first place. Now a court has to step in. A judge formally declares that you can no longer make your own decisions and appoints a guardian to make them for you. It's slower, costlier, and public, it comes with ongoing court supervision, and — most importantly — it takes the choice of *who decides* out of your hands entirely.

Here's the whole difference in one image. A power of attorney is *you* handing the keys to your life to someone you chose and trust. Guardianship is a *judge* deciding who gets those keys, after you've lost the chance to choose for yourself. Both end in the same place — someone deciding on your behalf. But one path keeps you in the driver's seat right up to the last moment; the other quietly removes you from the car.

GUARDIANSHIP IS A LAST RESORT — ON PURPOSE

Because guardianship strips away so much — often the right to decide where you live, what medical care you get, how your money is spent, sometimes even the right to vote — the law treats it as a *last resort.* Most states require that gentler options be considered first, and a broad coalition of experts, from the American Bar Association to federal disability agencies, has pushed hard in this direction.[4]

What are the gentler options? The very tools this book keeps returning to: a power of attorney, an advance directive — and a newer approach called **supported decision-making,** in which a person who needs help doesn't lose their rights at all. Instead, they keep the authority to decide their own life, and simply lean on a team of trusted people to help them understand the options and think things through — which, when you consider it, is exactly how most of us make big decisions anyway. The modern instinct is clear: help people keep their voice, not take it away.

This matters enormously for families caring for a loved one with a serious disability or advancing dementia. Guardianship is sometimes truly necessary, and when it is, it's an act of protection. But it should be the step you take when nothing gentler will do — not the first door you reach for.

THE ONE MOVE THAT CHANGES EVERYTHING

If there's a single thread running through this chapter, it's this: nearly all the pain in Tom's waiting room could have been prevented by one conversation, held years earlier, on an ordinary evening when nothing was wrong.

If Tom had named the person he trusted, his family wouldn't be wondering who's in charge. If Tom had once said out loud what mattered to him — what kind of life he'd want to fight for, and what he wouldn't — his daughter wouldn't be sobbing that she doesn't know. The choice would still be hard. But it would be *his,* carried faithfully by the people he loved, instead of a guess, or an argument, or a courtroom.

That one move — deciding, while you're well, *who* would speak for you and *what* you'd want — is the whole subject of this book's final chapter. For now, just know that it exists, that it's simple, and that it may be the greatest gift you ever give the people who would otherwise be left standing in that waiting room.

WHAT HAPPENED IN TOM'S FAMILY

Tom's family found their answer in an unlikely place.

On the third day, his daughter remembered something. Two summers earlier, after a movie about a man kept alive for years on machines, Tom had leaned back on the porch and said — half joking, the way people say the most important things — "If I ever end up like that, don't you dare keep me plugged in for years. Let me go."

Her brother remembered it the instant she said it. Their mother didn't; she had been in the kitchen.

It wasn't a document. It wouldn't have held up anywhere. But it was *Tom's own voice,* and the moment they heard it again, the argument in that waiting room changed shape entirely. They stopped asking each other what to do. They started asking what he had already told them.

They still had a terrible week. They still cried. But they made the decision together, and they made it the way Tom would have made it — and not one of them has ever had to lie awake since wondering whether they got it right.

Here's the part worth noticing, though: they got *lucky.* One offhand sentence, tossed off on a porch two summers before, happened to be overheard by the right person and remembered at the right moment. Most families don't get that.

And the whole point of the final chapter is that you don't have to leave it to luck.

WHAT THIS MEANS FOR YOU

If you're ever the one deciding for someone else, hold onto three things: look first for anything they wrote or said about their wishes; choose as *they* would choose, not as you would; and include the whole family while gently keeping everyone's eyes on the patient, not on their own grief.

And if you're thinking about yourself: don't wait. Name your person. Then actually talk to them — tell them what matters to you — so that if the day ever comes, they're not guessing.

THE GOOD NEWS

To need someone else to decide for you is one of the most vulnerable things that can happen to a human being. But it does not have to mean chaos, or courtrooms, or families torn in half over a hospital bed.

With just a little foresight, that frightening handoff can become something almost tender — your voice passing smoothly from your own hands into the hands of someone you chose and trust, exactly as you intended. And even in the hardest cases, notice the quiet beauty in how our system is built: try the gentlest path first, keep the person's own voice alive as long as humanly possible, take rights away only when there's truly no other way. That instinct reflects something worth believing in — that your right to shape your own life doesn't simply vanish the instant you can no longer speak. It lives on, in the wishes you shared and in the people who love you enough to honor them.

You can't always choose what happens to your body. But you *can* choose, starting today, whose hand will be holding yours when it matters most — and you can make sure they know your heart well enough to speak it. That's not losing control. That's the deepest kind of keeping it.

NOTES

[1] The standard model of surrogate decision-making follows a hierarchy: honor the person's own prior instructions (e.g., an advance directive) first; absent those, apply *substituted judgment* (choosing as the patient would have chosen, based on their values); and only when the patient's preferences cannot be known — or the patient never had decision-making capacity — apply the *best-interest standard.* See Beauchamp TL, Childress JF, *Principles of Biomedical Ethics*; and "Advance Directives and Substitute Decision-Making," *Stanford Encyclopedia of Philosophy.*

[2] Shalowitz DI, Garrett-Mayer E, Wendler D. "The Accuracy of Surrogate Decision Makers: A Systematic Review." *Archives of Internal Medicine.* 2006;166(5):493–497. Surrogates predicted patients' treatment preferences with approximately 68% accuracy.

[3] A healthcare power of attorney (also called a healthcare proxy or agent) is created by the individual in advance, without court involvement, and directs the agent to act on the person's own wishes. Guardianship, by contrast, is a court

proceeding initiated after a person is found to lack capacity. Requirements vary by state; consult your state's law or an elder-law attorney.

[4] Guardianship removes significant legal rights and is broadly regarded as a last resort, to be used only after less restrictive alternatives — such as powers of attorney, advance directives, and supported decision-making — have been considered. See U.S. Administration for Community Living, "Alternatives to Guardianship"; American Bar Association Commission on Law and Aging; and the U.S. Department of Justice Elder Justice Initiative.

CHAPTER EIGHT
BEING YOUR OWN ADVOCATE IN THE AGE OF AI

It's 2 a.m., and Rosa can't sleep. That afternoon a doctor gave her a diagnosis she'd never heard of, and now she's doing what almost all of us do: she's on her phone, searching.

The first site says her condition is manageable. The second says it's a death sentence. A forum is full of terrifying stories. A slick page promises a "natural cure the doctors won't tell you about" — for three easy payments. Finally she types her symptoms into an AI chatbot, which answers instantly, calmly, and with total confidence... and tells her something that, she'll learn next week, is partly wrong.

By 3 a.m. Rosa isn't informed. She's terrified, confused, and more lost than when she started.

If you've ever been Rosa — and almost everyone has — this chapter is for you. Because we live in an astonishing moment: never in human history have ordinary people had so much medical information at their fingertips. That's genuinely wonderful. It can save your life. But we're also drowning in *bad* information, and the single most valuable skill of our age is no longer *finding* information. It's telling the trustworthy from the toxic.

WHY THERE'S SO MUCH JUNK

Let's start by naming the problem honestly. The flood of health information online is so overwhelming, and so polluted with falsehood, that the World Health Organization gave it a name: an **infodemic** — too much information, mixed with false and misleading information, causing confusion, risky choices, and mistrust of the very experts trying to help.[1] On some health topics, studies have found that a huge share of what circulates on social media is simply wrong.

And here's the part that should make all of us more careful: the bad information doesn't just exist — it *travels faster than the truth.* In one landmark study of millions of online stories, researchers found that false information was about 70% more likely to be shared than true information.[2] Think about why. The truth is often boring, hedged, complicated. Lies can be made shocking, simple, and emotional — engineered to grab you by the collar. A calm, accurate fact rarely goes viral. "Doctors are hiding THIS from you!" spreads like fire.

So if you've ever felt that the scariest, most extreme claims are the ones that find you first — you're not imagining it. That's exactly how the system works.

THE NEW VOICE IN THE ROOM: AI

Into this world walks a powerful newcomer: the AI chatbot. Already, more than one in five adults have turned to AI to ask a health question. [3] And it's easy to see why — AI can be genuinely impressive. It's patient. It never makes you feel stupid for asking. It can translate baffling medical jargon into plain English in seconds. Some AI systems can even pass the same licensing exams that human doctors take.

But — and this is one of the most important "buts" in this whole book — AI has real and dangerous weaknesses that everyone using it for health needs to understand.

First, AI makes things up. Engineers call it "hallucination": the AI states false information with the exact same calm confidence it uses for true information. Recent audits of the most popular chatbots found they gave inaccurate or incomplete medical answers a substantial share of the time — and, alarmingly, sometimes *invented the scientific studies they cited,* producing references that don't exist.[4] The confidence is not a sign of correctness. AI sounds equally sure whether it's right or completely wrong.

Second, AI tends to tell you what you want to hear. Researchers have found that these systems can be "sycophantic" — leaning toward answers that agree with the assumptions in your question rather than correcting them. So if Rosa types, "Isn't it true that my condition means I'll die?", a chatbot may be nudged toward confirming her fear instead of calming it.

Third, AI doesn't know you. It has never examined your body, seen your history, or weighed your medications. It's a brilliant generalist speaking into the dark — with no idea who's on the other end.

None of this means AI is useless. Far from it. It means AI is a wonderful tool for *understanding and preparing* — and a dangerous one for *diagnosing yourself or making final decisions alone.* Use it to learn the questions. Never let it be the one who answers them for good.

A SIMPLE TOOLKIT FOR TELLING GOOD FROM BAD

Here's the empowering part: you don't need a medical degree to sort trustworthy information from garbage. You just need a few honest questions, and you can apply them to any website, video, post, or chatbot answer.

Who is saying it? Is there a real, named author with real credentials — a doctor, a hospital, a health agency? Or is it anonymous? Accountability matters.

Why are they saying it? Follow the money. Is this page ultimately trying to *sell* you something — a supplement, a miracle device, a subscription? A source that profits from your fear has already failed the trust test.

What's the evidence? Are there real studies and sources behind the claims, or just dramatic anecdotes and "I just know it works"? One person's story, however moving, is not evidence.

When was it written? Medicine changes. A confident article from many years ago may simply be out of date.

Does it fit the wider picture? If a single website claims something that *every* major medical organization contradicts, that's almost never a brave hidden truth being suppressed. It's almost always just wrong.

And learn to spot the red flags, because they repeat: miracle cures, "one weird trick," "what doctors don't want you to know," breathless all-caps urgency, conspiracy framing, and — always — something for sale.

On the other side, some sources have earned their trust by being accountable and evidence-based: government health resources like MedlinePlus and the CDC, major medical centers like the Mayo Clinic and Cleveland Clinic, and professional medical societies.[5] They're not flawless. But they show their work, they update, and they answer for what they publish. That's what trustworthy looks like.

THE REAL GOAL: A PARTNER, NOT A REPLACEMENT

Here's the reframe that ties this whole chapter together, and it reaches all the way back to what we said about informed consent: the point of becoming well-informed is *not* to become your own doctor. It's to become a great *partner* to your doctor.

The best medical outcomes don't come from a patient who Googled everything and stopped listening to professionals. And they don't come from a passive patient who nods at whatever they're told, either. They come from the powerful combination of an *informed patient* and a *competent clinician,* thinking together. You bring two things no chatbot and no website ever can: your knowledge of your own body, your life, and your values — and your questions. Your doctor brings training, experience, and the ability to actually examine you. Neither is complete without the other.

So use the good sources. Use AI carefully. Walk in prepared. Then say the most powerful sentence an empowered patient can say: "I read about this — does it apply to me?" That single question turns everything you found from a source of midnight panic into fuel for a real, grounded conversation.

Being your own advocate also means using your voice. It means asking questions until you understand. It means saying, out loud, "I don't follow — can you explain that again?" It means bringing a written list so your mind doesn't go blank, bringing a friend to a hard appointment so two sets of ears are listening, and never being afraid to seek a second opinion. Information gives you knowledge. Your voice turns that knowledge into advocacy.

WHAT THIS MEANS FOR YOU

The next time you're tempted to start down a 2 a.m. rabbit hole, try this instead:

Go to trustworthy sources first, and use AI to help you *understand* and to build a list of questions — not to hand you a diagnosis.

Run every important claim through the simple test: who's saying it, why, on what evidence, how recently, and does it match the wider medical consensus?

Treat a chatbot's confident answer as a *starting point to verify*, never as the final word — and remember it may be agreeing with your fears rather than correcting them.

Bring what you found to a real clinician who knows you, and ask the golden question: "Does this apply to *me*?"

Never, ever make a major medical decision on the say-so of a website or an AI alone.

WHAT ROSA DID NEXT

Rosa put the phone down at 3 a.m. and did not sleep well.

But the next morning she did something different. She went to *one* reliable source instead of twelve — a plain-language page from a major medical library — and read it slowly. It was less dramatic than anything she'd found at 2 a.m., and less certain, too. That turned out to be the point.

Then she used the AI again, but differently. Instead of asking "is this fatal," she asked it to explain three terms from her diagnosis in simple language, and to help her think of questions worth asking her doctor. It was genuinely good at that. She kept the questions and threw out its opinions.

She wrote eight questions on an index card. She asked her sister to come with her, because two sets of ears are better than one, and hers were not reliable that week.

The appointment ran long. Her doctor answered all eight questions. He told her that two of the things she'd read didn't apply to her at all, and that one did — but not in the way the website had made it sound. He corrected the chatbot on a point of fact. And he told her that one of her questions was a good one he hadn't thought to raise himself.

Rosa walked out with exactly the same diagnosis she'd walked in with. Nothing about her illness had changed.

What had changed was that she now understood it. And she was no longer facing it alone, at 3 a.m., with a glowing phone in a dark room. She was facing it with a plan, a doctor she could actually talk to, and her sister in the waiting room.

That's the whole difference. It isn't knowledge, exactly.

It's the end of being lost.

THE GOOD NEWS

We live in the most information-rich moment in the history of the human race. That is not something to be afraid of. Handled well, it's something closer to a superpower — one our grandparents, sitting silently in a doctor's office and never questioning a word, could only have dreamed of.

The terrified woman lost in the rabbit hole at 3 a.m. and the calm, prepared patient who walks into her appointment with a clear list of good questions are the *same person.* The only difference between them is a handful of skills — the ability to tell a trustworthy source from a toxic one, to use powerful new tools wisely instead of blindly, and to turn information into a real conversation with someone who knows both medicine and *you.*

You don't have to know everything. No one does, not even the doctors — that's what makes it a partnership. You just have to know how to find what's true, how to hold what's uncertain, and how to walk into that room as a full participant in your own care rather than a passenger.

That is what it means to be your own advocate. And in this astonishing, overwhelming, information-soaked age, it may be one of the most valuable things you can learn to be — for yourself, and for everyone you love.

NOTES

[1] World Health Organization, "Understanding the infodemic and misinformation in the fight against COVID-19" and related WHO resources. WHO defines an infodemic as an overabundance of information, including false or misleading information, that causes confusion, risk-taking behavior, and mistrust of health authorities. A WHO systematic review ("Infodemics and health misinformation," *Bulletin of the WHO,* 2022) found high rates of misinformation across health topics online.

[2] Vosoughi S, Roy D, Aral S. "The Spread of True and False News Online." *Science.* 2018;359(6380):1146–1151. False stories were roughly 70% more likely to be shared than true ones.

[3] Mayo Clinic, "Can you trust AI for health advice?" (2026), reporting that more than one in five adults worldwide use AI chatbots to ask health questions; and studies noting that some AI systems can achieve passing scores on the U.S. Medical Licensing Examination.

[4] Recent audits of widely used chatbots have documented frequent inaccurate or incomplete medical answers and fabricated ("hallucinated") citations, as well as a tendency toward "sycophancy" (favoring answers that agree with the user). See, e.g., the 2025 red-teaming audit of five popular chatbots reported in the *BMJ* and by CIDRAP (2025–2026), and Ayers JW, et al., "Comparing Physician and Artificial Intelligence Chatbot Responses to Patient Questions," *JAMA Internal Medicine,* 2023. Because AI systems change rapidly, current performance varies.

[5] For guidance on evaluating online health information, see MedlinePlus (U.S. National Library of Medicine), "Evaluating Health Information," and the U.S. Centers for Disease Control and Prevention. Reputable academic medical centers (e.g., Mayo Clinic, Cleveland Clinic) and professional medical societies are also generally reliable, accountable sources.

CHAPTER NINE
TAKING CONTROL BEFORE YOU HAVE TO

In February of 1990, a twenty-seven-year-old woman named Terri Schiavo collapsed in her home. Her heart stopped, her brain went too long without oxygen, and she never woke up again. She was left in what doctors call a persistent vegetative state — alive, but with no awareness, and no realistic hope of recovery.

And then something happened that turned a private tragedy into a national one. Terri's husband came to believe she would never have wanted to be kept alive this way, by a feeding tube, with no hope of return. Her parents believed the opposite — that she might recover, and that her life should be sustained. Both sides loved her. Both were certain they knew her heart. And because Terri had never written down a single word about what *she* would want, there was no way to answer the only question that mattered: *what would Terri have chosen for herself?*

So they fought. For years. The case wound through the Florida courts, then the state legislature, then the governor's office, then the United States Congress, then the President of the United States, and finally the Supreme Court. It played out on every television in America. Terri spent fifteen years in that condition. Her family was torn permanently in half. She finally died in 2005, at forty-one.

And here is the piece that should stay with you: nearly all of it was avoidable. One document — one quiet afternoon with a pen — could have prevented the entire fifteen-year ordeal.[1] Not the tragedy of her collapse. But the war that followed it.

This final chapter is about that pen. It's about the handful of simple documents that let you reach forward through time — past a stroke, past an accident, past your own last breath — and keep your voice, keep your control, and keep the people you love from having to guess, fight, and grieve all at once.

THE WHOLE BOOK HAS BEEN LEADING HERE

Look back at everything we've walked through. Consent. Weighing risk. Refusing treatment. Letting go. Who decides when you can't. Nearly every hard moment in this book becomes gentler, kinder, and less likely to tear a family apart with just a little preparation.

That preparation comes down to four documents. You don't need to be old. You don't need to be rich. You just need to be a person who would rather leave your loved ones a plan than a crisis. Let's take them one at a time, in plain words — each one answers a different question.

THE FOUR DOCUMENTS

A living will answers: "What do I want?"
A living will — also called an advance directive — is where you write down your wishes about medical care in case you can't speak for yourself: whether you'd want to be kept alive on machines, whether you'd want a feeding tube, whether you'd want to be resuscitated, and under what circumstances.[2] It is, quite simply, your own voice preserved on paper for the day you can't use it. This is the exact document Terri Schiavo didn't have — the one that would have ended the argument before it began.

A healthcare power of attorney answers: "Who speaks for me?"
We met this one back in the chapter on who decides. A healthcare power of attorney (also called a healthcare proxy or agent) names the specific person you trust to make medical decisions for you if you can't. Pair it with your living will and you've covered both bases: your living will says what you want, and your named person handles all the situations no document could have predicted. Together, they're the antidote to a court having to appoint a stranger — or a judge — to decide your most intimate matters.

A will answers: "Who gets what — and who raises my children?"
A last will and testament directs where your belongings and money go after you die. But for parents, it does something far more important than dividing up property: it lets you name who would raise your minor children if you couldn't. Without a will, both of those decisions fall to a court, decided by a rigid legal formula that may look nothing like what you would have chosen, through a slow and public process called probate. A will is you making those choices instead of a stranger in a courtroom.

A trust answers: "How is all of this managed?"
A living trust is a tool that holds and manages your assets. Its great advantages are that it can spare your family the delay, cost, and publicity of probate, and it can arrange for someone to manage your affairs smoothly if you become incapacitated. Not everyone needs a trust — a will is the essential foundation for most people — but for many families it's a powerful added layer of protection and privacy. This is the one worth asking a professional about for your particular situation.

Four documents. Four questions answered, in advance, by *you* — instead of by a court, a formula, or a family torn between grief and guessing.

The Strange, Sad Truth: Almost Nobody Does This

Here's what should stop you in your tracks. Despite how much these documents matter — despite the fact that everyone reading this will, someday, need someone to know their wishes — most people simply never make them.

Roughly two out of three American adults have no advance directive at all.[2] And when it comes to a basic will, only about one in four adults has even that.[3] We are, as a society, almost entirely unprepared for something that will happen to every single one of us.

Why? Not because we don't care. The surveys are painfully consistent: the number one reason people give is simply that they *haven't gotten around to it.* We put it off. We tell ourselves it's for the old, or the sick, or the wealthy. We flinch from thinking about our own mortality — which is deeply human, and completely understandable.

But here is the hard truth wrapped inside that flinch: **avoiding the paperwork does not avoid the event.** It only guarantees that when the event comes — and it comes to everyone — it arrives as chaos instead of as a plan. Terri Schiavo was twenty-seven and healthy the morning she collapsed. So was everyone who has ever been surprised by life. The document you keep meaning to make is only useful if you make it *before* you need it — and you almost never get to know when that is.

TWO GIFTS

When you finally sit down and do this, you give two gifts — and they are the two great themes this entire book has been circling from the very first page.

The gift to yourself is control. Your wishes, honored even when you can't voice them. Your values, still steering your care when you've gone silent. This is the deepest form of the idea we started with — that your life is *yours,* and that a real say in what happens to your own body is close to a human right. A living will and a healthcare proxy are that right, reaching forward into a future where you can't speak. They are your voice, refusing to be silenced by a stroke or an accident.

The gift to your family is peace. Remember how even loving family members guess a person's wishes correctly only about two-thirds of the time? These documents erase the guessing. No agonized wondering. No 3 a.m. arguments in a hospital hallway. No courtroom. No Schiavo-style war between people who all love you and all believe they're honoring you. Instead, you hand them clarity at the exact moment they'll need it most — the worst moment of their lives — so that they can spend their energy grieving and loving you, instead of fighting each other over you.

That is not a morbid gift. It may be one of the most generous things a human being can do for the people they love.

HOW TO ACTUALLY START

If this feels overwhelming, take a breath — it's smaller than you think, and you don't have to do it all at once.

Start with a *conversation.* Tell the person you trust most what matters to you — what kind of life you'd want to fight for, and what you wouldn't. That single talk does more good than most people imagine.

Then, the documents. Many are simpler and cheaper than you'd expect. Basic advance directive and healthcare proxy forms are often available for free through your state, your doctor's office, hospitals, or legal aid organizations. A will and a trust are worth doing with an attorney's help, but even that is far less costly than the probate mess and family strife their absence can cause. Name your healthcare agent. Write down your wishes. If you have children or property, make a will. Ask a professional whether a trust fits your situation.

And then — this part matters — revisit everything after any big life change: a marriage, a divorce, a new child, a new diagnosis. These documents are living things. Keep them current.

The single most important instruction in this entire chapter is also the simplest: *don't wait.* Not someday. This month. This week.

WHAT IT LOOKS LIKE WHEN SOMEONE DID THE WORK

We've spent this chapter on what happens when nobody wrote anything down. It's worth a moment on the opposite.

Imagine a woman named Eleanor. At seventy-one, she watched a friend's family tear itself apart over a hospital bed, and it frightened her enough that she went home and did something about it. It cost her one afternoon and two appointments. She filled out an advance directive saying plainly what she did and didn't want. She named her older daughter as her health care agent — not because she loved her more, but because that daughter was the steadiest under pressure, and Eleanor trusted her to honor her wishes even when it hurt to do it. She made a will. She talked with an attorney about a trust. And then she did the step almost everyone skips: she called both of her children and told them exactly what she had decided, and why.

Seven years later, Eleanor had a massive stroke.

Her family's week in that hospital was not painless. Nothing makes that painless. They cried in hallways. They held her hands. They grieved.

But look at everything that *didn't* happen. Nobody argued about who was in charge, because Eleanor had said. Nobody had to guess what she would have wanted, because Eleanor had written it down. Nobody went to court. No one's marriage strained. Her daughter, facing the hardest decision of her life, was not carrying the weight of *choosing* — she was carrying out instructions, and that is an entirely different burden. When she said, "This is what Mom wanted," it wasn't an opinion anyone could fight. It was Eleanor's own voice, still in the room.

And her son — who in another family might have been the one to object — had heard it years before, from his mother, in her own kitchen. There was nothing left to argue about.

Afterward they buried her, and then they went on being a family.

That last part is not a small thing. Ask anyone who has lived through the other version.

Eleanor's afternoon of paperwork didn't spare her a stroke. Nothing could have. What it spared was everything else: the guessing, the fighting, the courtrooms, and the lifelong ache of wondering whether you did right by someone you loved.

That is the whole offer of this chapter. Not that you can avoid the hard thing — but that you can decide, today, how much wreckage it leaves behind.

THE GOOD NEWS

Let's go back to where this book began — to that phone call at 3 a.m., and the questions that came flying at you in a hospital hallway when you had no answers ready. *Do you want us to do everything? What would she have wanted? Who has the authority to decide?*

This whole book has been built around two words: *Ask why.* Why do we choose what we choose. Why it matters so much who decides. And why we are so rarely, painfully ready.

This chapter is the answer to that last question — and the answer is that you don't *have* to be unready. That's the quiet miracle hidden in a few pieces of paper. You can be the person who, long before any crisis, calmly reached forward and took control. Who made sure your voice would carry even into rooms where you can't speak. Who made sure your wishes would be honored and your family would be spared. Who turned the worst day of their lives from a battlefield into something almost peaceful — a family gathered close, doing exactly what you asked, together.

That is not surrendering to death or disability. It is the opposite. It is refusing to let them take everything — refusing to let them steal your voice, your choices, and your family's peace along with your health. It is the last and deepest expression of the self-determination this book has been about from its very first page: *my life, my body, my choice* — carried all the way through to the end, and even a little beyond it.

You will not always be able to choose what happens to you. None of us can. But you can choose, starting today, that your voice will still be in the room when it matters most. You can choose to leave the people you love a map instead of a maze.

The best time to have done this was years ago. The second-best time is today.

Because in the end, this is what medical ethics — stripped of all its big words — has really been about the whole time: taking care of each other, as wisely and as lovingly as we can, all the way to the end of the story and past it. That care is one of the truest things human beings do.

And now, at last, you have everything you need to do it well.

NOTES

[1] The Terri Schiavo case (1990–2005) is widely cited in medical and legal ethics as the definitive illustration of what can happen when a person has left no written advance directive: the absence of any documented statement of her wishes led to a prolonged dispute among family members and years of litigation and legislative and political intervention. The details here reflect the documented public record of the case.

[2] For plain-language explanations of advance directives, living wills, and healthcare powers of attorney, see the U.S. National Institute on Aging, "Advance Care Planning: Advance Directives for Health Care." On prevalence: Yadav KN, Gabler NB, Cooney E, et al., "Approximately One in Three US Adults Completes Any Type of Advance Directive for End-of-Life Care," *Health Affairs* 2017;36(7):1244–1251 — found that about 37% of adults had completed any advance directive (about 29% a living will), meaning roughly two-thirds had none.

[3] Caring.com, *2025 Wills and Estate Planning Study* (conducted with YouGov), which found that only about one in four U.S. adults reported having a will, and that a majority had no estate-planning documents at all. Figures vary year to year; the persistent finding is that most Americans lack these documents.

APPENDIX
RESOURCES FOR PATIENTS AND FAMILIES

The chapters in this book were about facing hard moments well. This appendix is about not facing them alone. Below is a starting toolkit of trustworthy organizations, help lines, and free forms — grouped to match the topics of the book, so you can turn straight to what you need.

Two important notes before you begin. First, laws, phone numbers, and websites change over time, and many of these matters — especially advance directives, wills, guardianship, and minor-consent rules — **vary from state to state.** Always confirm the current details and your own state's requirements. Second, nothing here is a substitute for professional advice: for legal documents, consult a licensed attorney; for medical decisions, consult a qualified clinician who knows you. Think of this list as the first door, not the whole house.

IN A CRISIS — IMMEDIATE HELP

- **911** — for any medical emergency or immediate danger to life.
- **988 Suicide & Crisis Lifeline** — free, confidential, 24/7 support for anyone in emotional distress or crisis. **Call or text 988**, or chat at **988lifeline.org.** Veterans can press 1; for support in Spanish, text

AYUDA to 988. Services are available for those who are Deaf or hard of hearing.

- **SAMHSA National Helpline** — free, confidential, 24/7 treatment referral and information for mental health and substance use concerns. 1-800-662-4357 (1-800-662-HELP).

UNDERSTANDING YOUR RIGHTS AND YOUR CARE *(CHAPTERS 2–3: INFORMED CONSENT AND WEIGHING RISK)*

- **MedlinePlus** (U.S. National Library of Medicine) — plain-language, ad-free information on conditions, treatments, patient rights, and how to talk with your doctor. medlineplus.gov.
- **Your hospital's patient advocate or ombudsman** — most hospitals have one whose job is to help you understand your rights, resolve concerns, and get your questions answered. Ask at the front desk or patient-relations office.
- **A prepared question list** — before any major decision, bring written questions (What are my options, including doing nothing? What are the real numbers? What matters most for someone in my situation?) and don't hesitate to ask your clinician to explain things again, in plain words.

MENTAL HEALTH AND INVOLUNTARY TREATMENT *(CHAPTER 4)*

- **NAMI — National Alliance on Mental Illness** — information, support, and guidance for individuals and families navigating mental illness, crises, hospitalization, and treatment options. **HelpLine: 1-800-950-6264**, or text **"HelpLine" to 62640**, or **nami.org.** NAMI also has local affiliates in most communities.
- **SAMHSA's FindTreatment** — a searchable directory of mental health and substance use treatment providers. **findtreatment.gov.**
- **Treatment Advocacy Center** — for those wanting to understand their own state's civil-commitment and assisted-outpatient-treatment laws. **tac.org.**

FOR TEENS AND PARENTS *(CHAPTER 5)*

- **HealthyChildren.org** — the American Academy of Pediatrics' website for parents, covering children's and teens' health and how to involve young people in their own care. **healthychildren.org.**
- **Your pediatrician or family doctor** — the best first stop for questions about a teen's care, confidentiality, and when a young person can consent for themselves.
- **Your state or local health department** — because minor-consent and confidential-care rules differ by state, your local health department can explain what applies where you live.
- *(For parents of a child with a disability approaching adulthood, see "Supported decision-making" under Legal Help, below.)*

SERIOUS ILLNESS, HOSPICE, AND PALLIATIVE CARE *(CHAPTER 6)*

- **Get Palliative Care** — explains what palliative (comfort) care is, and helps you find a provider near you. **getpalliativecare.org.**
- **CaringInfo** (a program of the National Alliance for Care at Home) — free information on hospice and palliative care, serious-illness decisions, and caregiving. **caringinfo.org, 1-800-658-8898.**
- **The Conversation Project** — free, gentle guides for talking with the people you love about end-of-life wishes — including how to choose a health care proxy and how to be one. **theconversationproject.org.**

ADVANCE DIRECTIVES, LIVING WILLS, AND HEALTH CARE *PROXIES (CHAPTERS 7 AND 9)*

- **CaringInfo — free, state-specific advance directive forms** for all 50 states and D.C., with instructions. **caringinfo.org** (or call **1-800-658-8898** to have forms mailed).
- **AARP** — free printable advance directive forms by state, with guidance. aarp.org (search "advance directives").

- **Five Wishes** (from Aging with Dignity) — an especially user-friendly advance directive covering medical, personal, and spiritual wishes, available in many languages for a small fee. It also offers **Voicing My Choices** for teens and young adults and **My Wishes** for children. **fivewishes.org, 1-850-681-2010.**
- **PREPARE for Your Care** — free, step-by-step, video-guided help for thinking through and completing an advance directive, in English, Spanish, and other languages. **prepareforyourcare.org.**

WILLS, TRUSTS, GUARDIANSHIP, AND LEGAL HELP *(CHAPTERS 7 AND 9)*

- **Eldercare Locator** (a public service of the U.S. Administration for Community Living) — connects you to local services for older adults and families, including legal help and long-term-care planning. **1-800-677-1116, eldercare.acl.gov.**
- **Legal aid** — for free or low-cost legal help, including wills and directives for those who qualify. Find your local program at **lawhelp.org** or through the **Legal Services Corporation (lsc.gov).**
- **American Bar Association** — consumer resources on advance care planning and on supported decision-making as an alternative to guardianship, through its Commission on Law and Aging. americanbar.org.
- **Alternatives to Guardianship** (U.S. Administration for Community Living) — plain-language information on supported decision-making and other less-restrictive options. **acl.gov** (search "alternatives to guardianship").
- **For wills and trusts:** because these must follow your state's specific rules, consult a licensed **estate-planning or elder-law attorney** in your state. The Eldercare Locator and legal-aid links above can help you find one.

FINDING TRUSTWORTHY HEALTH INFORMATION *(CHAPTER 8)*

- **MedlinePlus** — reliable, plain-language health information from the National Institutes of Health, including guidance on **evaluating health information** online. **medlineplus.gov.**
- **Centers for Disease Control and Prevention** (CDC) — trusted public-health information. **cdc.gov.**
- **National Institute on Aging** — clear, reliable information on aging, caregiving, and advance care planning. **nia.nih.gov.**
- **Major academic medical centers** — such as the **Mayo Clinic** (mayoclinic.org) and **Cleveland Clinic** (my.clevelandclinic.org) — offer accurate, patient-friendly explanations of conditions and treatments.
- **Remember the test from Chapter 8:** before you act on anything you read or any answer from an AI, ask *who* is saying it, *why*, on *what evidence, how recently*, and whether it matches the wider medical consensus — then bring it to a clinician who knows you and ask, "Does this apply to me?"

This appendix is a starting point for information and support. It is not legal or medical advice, and the availability and details of these resources may change. For decisions that matter, verify the current information, check your own state's rules, and lean on qualified professionals — and on the people who love you.

www.ingramcontent.com/pod-product-compliance
Lightning Source LLC
LaVergne TN
LVHW050938210926
848482LV00013B/658
* 9 7 9 8 9 9 3 7 7 9 4 6 1 *